# 7 Steps to a Healthy Pregnancy

Dr. Erica Royal

# 7 Steps to a Healthy Pregnancy

Dr. Erica Royal

7 Steps to a Healthy Pregnancy

To my three beautiful children,

Erica, Frank, and Colin

who make motherhood a joy.

# Acknowledgements

This book was written with the kind and generous help of friends and family. Their encouragement and nudging motivated me to compile helpful basic information for families considering pregnancy.

My three children Erica, Frank, and Colin are my daily inspiration. They have shared their mother with thousands of patients over the years.

# Contents

A family is forever changed when a child is born. Pregnancy and childbirth are a part of a family's experience only a few times in a lifetime. It is a short season with a life changing result: a new baby. Special care during this

> Approximately 131 million women give birth in the world annually.

time is important to ensure the best outcome. Following are seven easy, but important, steps to consider for a healthy and happy pregnancy and a healthy baby. Pregnancy can be fun!

## Step 1: Get Healthy Before Conception

A healthy pregnancy starts before conception. The prospective mom and dad should review their medical, surgical and medication histories with their doctors.

Common factors that affect fertility in women include weight (overweight or underweight), hormone imbalance, certain medical conditions, smoking, alcohol, and hazardous exposure.

Ideally, if any medical problems are present both partners and their doctors should have good control of the issues before conception. For example, if thyroid disease in women is not well controlled, it can interfere with conception. Diabetes with consistently high or abnormal blood sugar can lead to birth

defects and poor outcomes for baby and

mom. Well-controlled diabetes can

significantly minimize, if not eliminate, some

of these risks.

Certain medicines

are not safe in

> Common factors that affect fertility in men include smoking, alcohol, drugs (illegal and prescription), toxic exposure, certain medical conditions, and too much heat.

pregnancy. Usually, however, safe

alternatives exist. Expectant parents should

consult their doctors about switching to these

safe alternatives.

Mom must ensure that her vaccines are up to

date because once pregnant, her immune

system is more vulnerable, and she cannot

have certain vaccines. For example,

chickenpox can lead to maternal and fetal

death if acquired during pregnancy.

Men should also consult with their doctors.

Diabetes, certain medications, toxic

exposures, and a history of certain childhood

diseases can significantly affect the health

and quality of sperm.

Lastly, don't smoke!

Smoking can decrease fertility for both men and women. Alcohol consumption can too.

That goes for both

parents.

## Step 2: Get Early Prenatal Care

Getting prenatal care early allows for

accurate dating of

the pregnancy,

access to more

testing to

> Between 75% and 85% of couples will conceive in the first year that they try.

diagnose problems, and early intervention.

Also mom can learn from her doctor what she

should expect during her pregnancy. She

then has repetitive opportunities to ask her

medical team questions (medical and

nonmedical) as the stages of her pregnancy

progress.

Mom will have a partner invested in the

health of her pregnancy in addition to her

friends and family members. This support

contributes to a positive experience during

the pregnancy and birth.

Healthy parents contribute to a healthy baby!

## Step 3: Keep Prenatal Appointments

The numerous doctor appointments during pregnancy can seem mundane and unnecessary; however, subtle changes occur with mom and baby daily. A lurking abnormality can be often be detected during a routine appointment, early enough to be treated. Also, these appointments are great opportunities to reassure other members of the family (especially dad) that mom and baby are OK. Dads worry more than might be expected. Other children can participate during appointments too. I let older siblings hold the Doppler ultrasound instrument to hear the baby's heartbeat on mommy's tummy. This helps the family bond with the

baby.

Show up for appointments and remember to

ask questions during visits!

## Step 4: Exercise

Proper exercise is great for the pregnant

mom. It also makes

her feel better.

Certain types

Pregnant women are advised to
consult their doctors before beginning
any exercise program.

of exercises specific to pregnancy can help

quell pregnancy discomforts and help with

labor too.

Too much weight gain, which can cause

increased risk to mom and baby, can be

prevented with

Studies suggest that a mother's

exercise during pregnancy enhances

a child's brain development and can

exercise. Also,

reduce the risk of cardiovascular

mom's return to

disease over the child's lifetime.

normal

postdelivery occurs more quickly with proper

exercise. Keep moving!

## Step 5: Get Proper Sleep and Rest

Many women are used to burning the candle at both ends. This is not a good idea when pregnant because of a complex mix of hormones, physical changes, and sometimes emotional changes. Sleeping well helps a pregnant mom manage these complex changes better. Things like depression can be exacerbated with a lack of sleep. Remember too that when the baby comes, sleep may be minimized.

Rest and sleep well, mom. You have a magnificent excuse!

## Step 6: Eat Well and Drink Plenty of Water

Eating well does not mean eating large portions, frequently referred to as eating for two. Mom will, however, be eating for her health and the baby's health. Consuming generous helpings of fruits and vegetables and staying away from junk food is always a good idea.

> Gestational diabetes arises during pregnancy and results from the effect of changing hormones. It usually resolves itself after delivery.

Hypertension, gestational diabetes, fetal exposure to harmful bacteria in certain foods can be lurking complications. In general, small frequent meals are best! Mom must review special dietary concerns with her doctor.

Water consumption is very important also. Too little hydration can lead to premature contractions, not enough fluid around the baby, and swelling. Yes, swelling. If mom doesn't drink enough water, the body holds on to fluid, and she scan swell as a result. Drink up, ladies! No alcohol, of course.

## Step 7: Take Your Vitamins

Significant and ongoing research goes into the production of prenatal vitamins. Prenatal vitamins have some ingredients in doses that can be life changing for mom and baby. Folic acid helps to prevent neural tube defects in baby. Iron helps prevent maternal anemia, which can lead to extreme fatigue and danger at delivery if there is significant blood loss. DHA has been linked to a decreased incidence of premature labor and higher IQs in children. I knew my children were smarter than I am!

Pop those pills ... well, vitamins!

## Final Note

Most importantly, enjoy pregnancy! I hope the

above steps empower moms and dads and

help them have a healthy and pleasant

journey.

Be well, mommy!

# About the Author

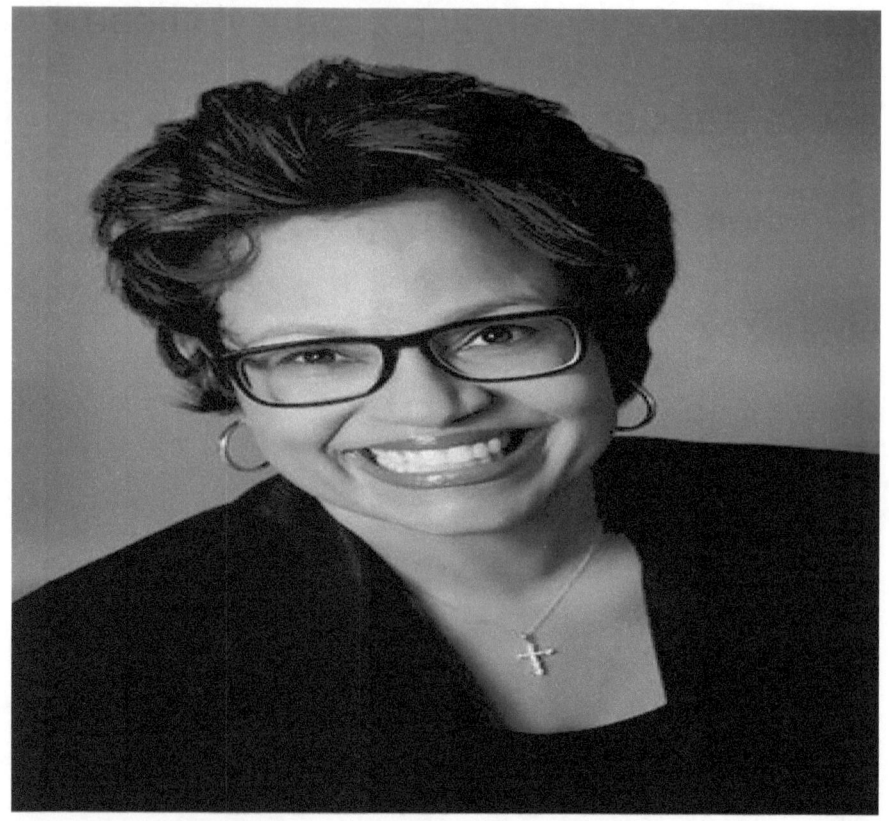

Dr. Royal is a proud mother of three beautiful

children: Erica, Frank, and Colin.

She is also a board certified

obstetrician/gynecologist who has been in

private practice for over 14 years.

Dr. Royal has served as vice-chairman and chairman of the OB/GYN department at Henrico Doctors Hospital where she is currently chief of staff elect.

Dr. Royal's professional and personal motto is "Let's live well together."